An Introduction to
Medical Ethics

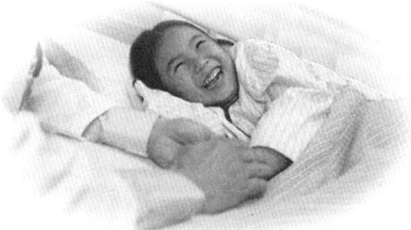

patient's interest first
Second Edition

An Introduction to
Medical Ethics

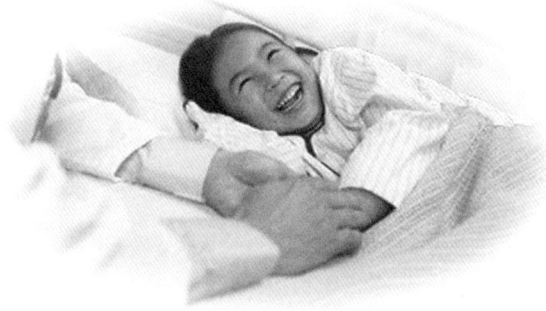

patient's interest first

Second Edition

Arthur SM Lim

W⊖ World Scientific

NEW JERSEY · LONDON · SINGAPORE · BEIJING · SHANGHAI · HONG KONG · TAIPEI · CHENNAI

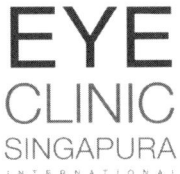

An Eye Clinic Singapura International publication with
World Scientific Publishing

Published by
World Scientific Publishing Co. Pte. Ltd.
5 Toh Tuck Link, Singapore 596224
USA office: 27 Warren Street, Suite 401-402, Hackensack, NJ 07601
UK office: 57 Shelton Street, Covent Garden, London WC2H 9HE

An Introduction to Medical Ethics:
Patient's Interest First, 2nd ed.

ISBN 978-981-279-304-1 (pbk)
World Scientific Publishing Co. Pte. Ltd.

"Let us battle for patient's interest and not for more rules, more regulations."

Preface

There is a need for a simple introduction to medical ethics, a topic which is not well-taught. With the advice of designers and editors, I manage to keep the volume small and readable, as well as emphasize the fundamental issues of ethics with the hope that this small publication will be a stimulus to students and young doctors to remember the importance of medical ethics when treating patients.

Arthur SM Lim

Introduction

What is Ethics?

Ethics is a social concept of good behavior. It is a collective concept that evolves gradually, usually over years, as a result of interaction between individuals living or working together.

Over the course of time, based on a common interest, an approved trend becomes established.

As such, apart from moral sanctions and personal disapproval, there is little to ensure that a collective concept is obeyed.

> Ethics is therefore a concept with no compelling force other than popular opinion.

In that sense, it is more akin to conscience than to law. In law, graded penalties are devised to suit the severity of any offense. On the other hand, ethics is seldom enforceable with the threat of punishment and conformity is achieved through the force of group opinion.

The Ethical Code and Medical Registration

Medical ethics is governed by the collective opinion and behavior of the medical profession. It has no legal standing in most situations, other than the disapproval of colleagues.

> However, with legal powers granted under the Medical Registration ordinance, medical ethics has, in fact, become more than just medical group opinion.

In many countries, members of the profession are required by law to be registered. In such circumstances, ethical conformity can be enforced by the threat of de-registration.

Nevertheless, it is still different from the law in that the penalties are confined to warnings, suspensions and de-registrations. Only recently were fines introduced. In contrast, criminal law embodies punishment ranging from corrective confinement, imprisonment and fines to corporal punishment and capital sentences.

Furthermore, the rules and regulations of medical ethics are not set out in writing. The professional bodies may publish ethical guidelines for information, which include a few precedents from previous inquires. This is unlike the law which sets out in considerable detail the infringements and the severity of punishments.

> *...the rules and regulations of medical ethics are not set out in writing. The professional bodies may publish ethical guidelines for information...*

Therefore the profession has been largely unregulated and a question to consider is whether there is a need for a profession to have its own ethics? Is the law of the land inadequate?

> While altruism is praiseworthy, it requires unconditional benevolence which goes against human nature.

Self-sacrificing altruism cannot be maintained except by a few. It would therefore be unrealistic for the profession to claim that it can expect such altruism from its members.

It is interesting to observe that self-regulatory activity is adopted by many other respectable bodies such as the clergy and the legal profession.

The Power of Medical Knowledge

The concept that "knowledge is power" has been highlighted and it is well-accepted that power can rule and destroy.

> We fear knowledge because we see it as a source of power which can damage if it is not exercised under rigid self-discipline.

It is too readily assumed that a professional man by virtue of his special knowledge will be charitable and benevolent. He can be a source of harm.

Regulation by legislation is inadequate by nature of its operation. It cannot be of much value in prevention by basing on acts already committed and detected. Hence, what is

Hence because the doctor's skill either saves lives or causes deaths, he relies on a code of ethics to prevent his own weakness. Society depends on the doctors' code in order to prevent deviant professionals from becoming a threat.

needed is not a punitive measure — for there would first have to be victims. What is required is a preventive measure before the problem materializes, for ethics represents a regulation of desire even before an act has taken place.

From the community's viewpoint, an ethical code ensure that specialized knowledge was being used for the benefit of patients and society.

It is essential that harm to patients must be prevented.

... a clear indication that the interest of the patient is foremost.

The medical ethical code, therefore, must ensure that medical service is being dispensed efficiently, with a clear indication that the interest of the patient is foremost.

Ethics Important for Practising Clinicians

Medical ethics is usually initiated by practising clinicians. This is why it puts so much stress on the aspect of patient-doctor relationship such as professional confidentiality, as well as adultery between the doctor and his patient.

The trend of modern life is towards greater collective efficiency. With the rise of community interest some doctors would be community physicians rather than doctors of individuals. There must be differences between the two.

For example, although professional confidentiality demands that a person's secret be kept confidential when a doctor learns about it through his practice, the community frequently compels the release if such information on the basis of the benefit to society. The doctor now finds himself in a conflict of having two masters to serve, the patient and the community.

History

In primitive societies, the doctor was regarded as a supernatural figure capable of influencing the mysterious forces of nature.

Because he was thought to have knowledge ordinary mortals had no access to, people conferred on him an absolute authority. Such authority of doctors no longer exists in modern societies. The last twenty years, in particular, have witnessed the growth of patients' rights.

Doctors are no longer in a position to insist that their acts be immune from questioning by society. Society has made them accountable.

Two thousand years ago, Hippocrates formulated an oath that provided an ethical standard for physicians.

This oath creates high ideals. But it was not until the first two decades of this century that medical councils were formed to institutionalize these and regulate the professional conduct of medical practitioners.

> Far from seeing these medical council as an intrusion on their individual freedoms, most doctors have accepted them freely.

Review of Doctors' Conduct

Doctors recognize that if they are to function as members of a credible profession, their conduct must be reviewed and reformed.

A skilled surgeon without ethics can be dangerous. His knowledge and skills are powerful weapons and we expect him to use them to save lives and help his fellowmen. However, these weapons can do harm if he has poor ethics and wrong values.

All the As — Alcohol, Abortion, Advertisement and Adultery can embarrass a doctor's ethics. For example, a doctor's alcoholism cannot be allowed to diminish or affect his clinical ability and judgment. A doctor may have his mistress made his patient, but he cannot have his patient as his mistress.

The Super and Postindustrial Economy in Singapore
How will ethics be changed?

Numerous thinkers have made predictions about the world's future. Perhaps the most optimistic is the remarkable futurologist Herman Kahn, who in 1977 declared: *"200 years from now, we expect almost everywhere they will be numerous, rich and in control of the forces of nature. Emergence of sup industrial economies (where enterprises are extraordinary large) to be followed soon by the post-industrial economies (where the task of producing the necessities of life has become trivially easy)."*

If Herman Kahn's prediction come true, Singapore will emerge with a super industrial economy, followed by a post-industrial one. The emergence of super and post-industrial technology in medicine has already begun, as can be seen in the introduction of operating microscopes, lasers, CAT scans and magnetic imaging.

Twenty years from now we will witness even more esoteric technology. Our successors will consider ordinary what we think of today as amazing! They may even view us as ignorant, foolish and hopelessly crude.

Medicine in Cities

Undoubtedly, the future for medicine is bright.

Today, medicine has become a controversial and an emotional, political and financial issue. With this new ethical issue will emerge.

When societies were largely rural and medical knowledge primitive, health care was mainly a local issue. When societies become largely urban and medical knowledge proliferating, health care becomes a concern to everyone.

> For when people live in close proximity, it is not possible to ignore the sick and when sophisticated technology is available, it is not possible to deny this to those who cannot afford.

The future of medicine and its ethics is complicated and will be determined not by doctors alone and ethics will be influenced by various forces — political, economic, social, technological — more powerful and embracing than the profession itself.

Ethics and Medical Advances

Because of advances in technology, it is now possible for doctors to carry out procedures which for decades we could only dream about. Test tube babies, organ transplantation already exist. Other procedures, like determining the genetic make-up of our off-spring, or cloning ourselves, pose grave ethical problems.

This development will lead to many interesting questions. When is a person dead? In the past, the heartbeat was the basic criteria, obviously this has changed.

... the genetic make-up of our off-springs or cloning ourselves pose grave ethical problems. When is a person dead? In the past, the heart beat was the basic criteria; obviously, we can no longer do so.

The long queue for transplants has forced doctors to make life and death decision about patients for non-clinical reasons. Should doctors refuse, for example, to perform foetal tissue transplant if it discovered that the potential recipient paid a woman to abort her baby for that purpose? What is the difference between a foetus obtained from a miscarriage and one obtained from an abortion? And who decides?

Medical ethics, obviously, will have to grapple with the challenges of tomorrow.

Social Transformation

In Singapore, rapid social transformation has led the government to modify some of our traditional ethical customs through legislation. Consider, for example, the legalizing of abortion.

The considerable disagreement within the medical profession as to the wisdom of legalizing abortion was not surprising. It must be remembered that members of the medical profession have for long been taught that it was criminal to perform abortions. The Hippocratic Oath, an ethical guide for the profession for centuries, states unequivocally: *"I will not give to a woman pessary to produce abortion."* When a new law transformed what was a serious professional, ethical and criminal offense into a social obligation, it was not surprising that it was received with great reservation by the medical profession.

Another example to consider is the change in the Medical Registration Act which allows the state to remove from the medical register, qualified practitioners who are found guilty of committing offenses not necessarily medical in nature. The law, for example, allows the Medical Council to remove a medical practitioner from the Register if he fails to fulfill the bond he has signed.

The above illustrations should not be interpreted as criticisms of the changes; instead, they should serve to emphasize the importance of understanding the social transformation of Singapore, and the need for us, as doctors, to expect further laws which will greatly affect our professional practice and our ethics.

Political, social economic and technological forces will continue to influence the ethics of medical practice.

These changes in the coming decades will create controversies. But doctors must always remember that their patients' interest must always be foremost.

Teaching Medical Ethics — or Punishment!

"Facts and knowledge can be communicated but wisdom and ethics cannot."

One of the problems facing Singapore is that medical ethics was not adequately taught at the university. The teaching of medical ethics to undergraduates is vital to impress ethical ideas upon the younger generation at an impressionable stage of their career. University teachers should not only teach the clinical signs and symptoms, diagnosis and management, but also discuss ethical controversies during clinics.

In a society of rapidly changing values where the marketplace increasingly intrudes into our professional lives, a deliberate approach to ethical questions will help us think. It is also important that practising doctors should hold forums and discuss medical ethics regularly.

It is impossible to lay down ethical rules for every situation. Medicine continually poses new and unexpected ethical new issues and our ethical positions have to be constantly re-examined in the light of changing values.

Medical practitioners must continue to reflect on ethics throughout their careers. This will constantly remind them of their responsibilities and will help them follow the ethical code as a philosophy that is adhered to by honorable professionals and not simply out of the fear of punishment.

> We must remember that ethics is not just
> a set of rules; it is a way of life.

We cannot maintain a way of life in the face of numerous challenges without re-examining our conscience repeatedly. That, ultimately, is a major burden of being a doctor in an increasingly complex world.

> The least desirable method is through
> the use of punishment.

It is the least desirable because ethics and moral consciousness are, in the final analysis, a personal responsibility. No amount of discipline, policing and punishment can maintain high standards if a concept of good behavior is not already present in the consciousness of individuals. However, in any society or in any profession, there are always a few who do not understand or who do not wish to understand the importance of maintaining a high standard of medical ethics. The profession has no alternative but to deal with these members.

If the profession does not regulate itself, the reputation of the profession as a whole will suffer, and the government or legislature will be forced to act on behalf of the public.

The necessity of regulation, however, should not lead us to forget that medical ethics is fundamentally the doctor's personal outlook on his professional life.

Although medical ethics may have little relation to the doctor's technical training or his diagnostic skills, it has a significant influence on the degree of success he attains in his relationship with his colleagues and in his handling of his patients.

The ethical code is more than just a set of rules. It is a philosophy; a philosophy which we will do well to look upon as a guide to professional behavior, a means of reflecting upon our duty to our fellow men.

Arthur SM Lim

What makes a good doctor?

This is probably one of the most important
questions asked in Singapore today.

Is a good doctor measured by how much he knows?

Does it depend on his skills? Or his ethics?

Through the ages, many have described doctoring as

the **noblest of professions**.

There are good reasons to do so.

A doctor treats the sick, rich or poor;

a doctor responds to need and help day or night.

A good doctor is dedicated, even without financial

returns; he consoles the sick with compassion.

Some doctors extend their skills to other countries

without financial reward. A doctor is also a teacher

and helps others through research.

A doctor does not only deliver quality care – *he promotes excellence.*

Most importantly, good doctors are kind. Kindness and compassion in a doctor combined with skills and knowledge are the measure of the noblest of the professions. Some past philosophers, especially Hindus, even equate a good doctor to a god.

In general, a good doctor will act according to his moral conscience and will follow the ethical code, not because he has to, but because **it is right**.

A major concern

of our students who aspires to take up doctoring

these days, is what the future holds for medicine.

I have often been asked about the prospects of

doctors. It is my belief that a good doctor will

have an excellent future in Singapore

Let me explain...

When I was a medical student,

Singapore was a very poor country. The mood then was different. We were not concerned with making money. We wanted independence for our country, freedom from British colonial rule, freedom to determine our own destiny. Through our people's hard work and toil, we have become affluent and we have become a wealthy, developed nation.

The passing from one stage to another

is a wonderful period – a period of transition – and

should be greeted with great optimism.

It is a period which comes with an opportunity

of a lifetime – the unique task of transforming

the medical destiny of Singapore.

The changes are necessary because we have **become** *wealthier*, *our patients* more demanding.

We need to communicate and elevate standards.

The changes in medicine are taking place in every country but with great differences. The changes the West have to cope with include a worsening situation in their health care system. In the United States, the government has to control health expenditure because health services now account for 16% of the GNP.

Research grants have been cut in Europe and United States.

What of **medicine** in Singapore?

Singapore

is now perhaps in the most important

phase of establishing itself as an

international medical hub.

We have the infrastructure, we have well-trained and
highly intelligent doctors, and we have an efficient
Ministry of Health.

Singapore has never been more

stable politically

or more prosperous.

Singapore has become one of the world's most advanced centers of commerce, finance, information technology, education, culture and communication.

What of medicine?

Once we have identified **the best doctors**, it would be wrong not to allow them a free hand to develop their skills to the maximum with little interference from administrators.

The greatest attraction for our top specialists to excel is the opportunity to become even better.

Although it is not always possible to have unity amongst intelligent and enthusiastic doctors, we must strive at it. As the people who run the famous Cleveland Clinic put it,

"to have unity is to succeed."

Today, we have to stay competitive.

If we do not improve our standards, our training,

and monitor the quality of care, whilst it may be all

right in the short term, it will not

benefit us or Singapore in the long run.

To achieve excellence,
we must attract the most mentally
agile, the most able, and the most
dedicated of our specialists to
play a major role in
establishing Singapore as
a leading medical center.

We must identify our
brightest young doctors

at an early age for rapid training and

accelerated promotion.

If Singapore can achieve higher standards than
the surrounding countries, with standards equal to,
if not better than those in Britain, Australia,
and America, we can become a major tertiary
referral center. Our patients will not be just
the 4.0 million Singaporeans but will include
hundreds and thousands of patients from
overseas as well.

How is an excellent reputation created? How do we recognize medical excellence?

Good results are essential.

Doctors must have knowledge,

skills and experience.

Experience does not mean that they have to be old.
It means that doctors have to learn every
procedure carefully, step by step, especially
the complicated procedures, to attain perfect results.

Unfortunately, some young surgeons think that as soon as they seen or assisted in a surgical procedure once or twice, they can perform the operation effectively. This can be disastrous.

Experience would mean that doctors need to follow a good leader, a good doctor or a good surgeon, and to follow him through 10, 20 or 100 procedures.

The identification
of a first rate doctor is essential.

Young doctors will learn his good habits and
techniques, why he has fewer complications and why
his results are almost perfect. This is the only way
to ensure that the doctors in the next generation
will be just as good and hopefully even better.

It is well known

that an hour with a skilled and
wise master surgeon is worth
a month of study.

On the other hand, if a doctor follows a second rate surgeon, he will end up as a third rate surgeon.

It is important to know **values**.

Some doctors may wonder what they stand to gain financially. Financial matters are important but must be placed in the proper perspective.

Good doctors will have a very interesting and excellent

future but not in terms of earning a lot of money.

Doctors who want to become multi-millionaires

rapidly should leave their medical studies and

join the stock exchange or go into business.

Good doctors

will be financially comfortable and well respected.

Income will be good but not spectacular.

Their patients, whose interest

must always be foremost,

are occasionally wealthy, but usually poor.

They can never be good doctors if they are capable of turning away a patient suffering from a complicated illness, simply because he is unable to pay.

I am happy to say that in my 30 years of practice, I have not turned away a single patient with a major blinding problem on the grounds of finance.

There were occasions in which I paid for the patient's hospitalization and other medical costs.

Doctors must always remind themselves that their

skills are only of value if used to

help and comfort

their patients.

New technology,

which is essential for advancement, will continue to

be introduced in Singapore. This is exciting — doing

lung operations through 2 cm incisions, taking out

the gall bladder with small incisions. However, we

have to be careful and evaluate the outcome.

The latest is not always the best.

There is a dark side to new technology.

These new techniques can cause serious complications.

So until the doctor has been properly trained and

is sure, he must not move too quickly into

doing these new procedures.

I was very distressed when a young ophthalmologist asked me:

"How can I learn new techniques if I do not practise on my patients?"

"Practise?" I asked, horrified, "On the eyes of your patients? Why don't you use the laboratory?"

"But that's not the same," came his answer.

"Anyway, the 'Learning Curve' is quite accepted around this world."

This is just one example of a serious erosion
of professional ethics that has been brought
about by the overeager acceptance of
new technology and procedures.

A good doctor must know that before he carries out

any procedure, the age-old medical adage must prevail:

"First of all, do no harm."

Even as we explore new medical technologies,

our main concern should be the welfare of our patients,

not the development of our skills or

the advancement of our research interest

or better financial returns.

Always remember,
the interest of our patients must
be foremost in our minds.

A good doctor must maintain healthy relationships with his colleagues, his patients and the society in which he lives and serves.

A doctor's

relationship with his colleagues

is one of the most important of his professional life.

It is essential that doctors regard their colleagues with fraternal respect and in a setting of keen professional competition, avoid the temptation of disparaging each other. Intra-professional jealousy has escalated in modern cities like Singapore, where hundreds of doctors and specialists work in the same hospitals and medical centers, interacting for the benefit of their patients.

Respecting their teachers

and acknowledging and praising

the excellence of their colleagues

are issues doctors should address.

The senior doctors must teach

the young doctors all they can and hope that their

younger colleagues become better than they are.

The students and younger doctors

must appreciate and acknowledge the opportunities

given to them so that they may even surpass

the skills of their professors.

In ancient society, the doctor was regarded as a supernatural figure as he grappled with the serious and mysterious **forces of disease and health.**

In the information age,

the situation has changed. In contrast to

the acceptance of professional authority in the first

half of last century, a growing public concern

amongst patients for

their rights has emerged in the last decade.

As our patients become more affluent and educated, they will be more demanding. In many ways, this is good as such demands encourage health care providers to give the best service.

I must emphasize that

a good doctor/patient relationship is essential for good patient care.

I always strive to maintain this relationship,

and I feel sad when a patient's relationship

with me deteriorates, as I would experience

difficulty in managing that patient well.

For this reason it is important to have good and

clear communication with a patient.

The public, in its enthusiasm for rights,

should remember that the patient whose life

is in danger; who is in danger of losing

the sight of his only eye; who is in need of being

relieved of pain and suffering is less concerned with

his rights, but in having a good and compassionate

doctor who will do his utmost to help him.

I have already explained that

it is most important to ensure that the

patient's interest
is foremost.

No government will take a doctor
seriously if he is only interested
in his own welfare and disregards
the interest of society.
We must remember that the
medical profession, although
important, represents only a
small part of the multitude of
the problems that a nation faces.

As society becomes more complex, the doctor's role in treating individual patients often comes into conflict with the requirements of the community.

A well-known problem faced by doctors is professional secrecy.

We all know that a patient's medical condition

is confidential.

How do doctors respond to a patient who is a very good pilot, but has epilepsy and may endanger the lives of passengers? How should doctors deal with a patient with venereal disease or worse, AIDS?

Is it not for the patient, as a responsible person, to
inform those associated with him of his condition?
Will it not deter a patient from seeking
medical treatment unless he is assured that his secret
will only be shared with his doctor?

It seems to me that when the medical practitioner feels
that a patient's condition poses a threat to others,
he faces a dilemma as he also has a moral obligation
to make that danger known.

As societies become more complex, doctors have to
work with the requirements of their society.
Their responsibility today is not just to
their patients as individuals, but also to society.

Some important current issues of medical ethics:

It would be wise for doctors not
to ignore the national problem of
costs for good health care.

It is clear that in our inflationary
society with an aging population,
costs will spiral.

Good, affordable patient care is one of the most challenging issues facing doctors, the public and the government. In general, it appears sound to have direct financing from source as this can help reduce unnecessary expenditure.

A major weakness is that for chronically ill patients

who need long periods of medical care,

the costs can be enormous and the savings

of such patients are easily exhausted.

Who is going to pay?

The medical professions in several countries generated considerable controversy when they liberalized advertisement.

A strong argument in favor of liberalizing information on the achievements of doctors is that if the excellence of their work is not known to the public, the image of doctors can deteriorate.

This has become important as publicity on doctors

is frequently negative, highlighting punishment

by the Medical Council or

in a court of law. And if publicity on advances

in medicine is repeatedly made only

by overseas doctors, the reputation of

local doctors will suffer.

Furthermore, if Singapore desires to be an international medical center, our doctors must not only be excellent, but shown to be excellent.

There are of course problems.

Who decides? Who can advertise? In what way?

How often? **What** if the statements are untrue?

I believe that we should review this controversial issue carefully and introduce safeguards — the most important of which is to ensure that statements made are true.

If nothing is done soon, one of the unfortunate results

will be the insidious decline of the image of doctors.

Doctors are already occasionally unjustly

accused of being uncaring, questionable,

dishonest and unethical money grabbing professionals.

This image is of course untrue.

But unless we act to stop this,

all doctors may slide into this sad and

slippery decline of our reputation.

Unfortunately, there are the black sheep.

We must expose them and act against them.

In conclusion,

I must again emphasize that above anything else,

the ethical principle which holds that

the patient's interest must always be foremost

should be upheld as the chief consideration

in the doctor's relationship with his patients.

We must always remember that
a doctor's true value is the good
he does for his patients and
his fellowmen.